THE STRETCHING HANDBOOK

Your Guide to Avoiding Sports Injury & Improving Athletic Performance !

BRAD WALKER
Exercise Scientist & Sports Trainer

WHAT ARE THE EXPERTS SAYING ABOUT

THE STRETCHING HANDBOOK ?

"The Stretching Handbook by Brad Walker provides a comprehensive guide to the art of stretching. The detailed photographic catalogue of stretching exercises serves as an easy to follow reference guide for athletes and coaches alike."

Wayne Pearce
Coach - Balmain Tigers RLFC

"Stretching is an important part of any exercise program to help prevent injury and to increase flexibility. The Stretching Handbook is a clear, concise guide to stretches for all areas of the body."

Bob Fulton
Coach - Manly Sea Eagles RLFC & Australian Team Coach

"The acceptance of the importance of flexibility and stretching for sport is commonplace, but appropriate and accessible information for athletes and coaches to use, is not always easy to find. The Stretching Handbook is designed to be a very portable and quick reference for athletes and coaches rather than an academic reference. To this end it is a very practical text with concise chapters written in an easy to read manner but without being punctuated by research findings or scientific references."

"Overall, The Stretching Handbook is well laid out, user friendly and very suitable for athletes and developing coaches. It is a welcome addition to the limited number of texts which deal with stretching for sport."

Angela Calder
Performance Consultant - Australian Institute of Sport

"An excellent, important guide to optimum health and peak performance. Read, learn, implement and enjoy the benefits of wellness and enhanced quality of life."

Dr Denis Waitley, (PhD)
Author & Past Chairman - US Olympic Committee

"A thoroughly professional and comprehensive book on a subject that previously was very much neglected. It will play an important role for coaches and athletes in preparation for their specific sports. The Stretching Handbook is a must for anybody involved in the health and fitness industry."

Tony Green
Strength & Conditioning Coach - Gold Coast Chargers RLFC

"The first publication to thoroughly cover the importance of stretching to improve performance, avoid injury and assist in recovery. A vital part of any athletes complete conditioning program."

Craig Starcevich (B.Ed.)
Fitness Co-ordinator - Brisbane Lions Football Club

"The Stretching Handbook is a useful resource for all coaches. The photographs and explanations are clear and concise. A much needed resource."

Janet Bothwell
National Director of Coaching - Netball Australian

"Overall I believe The Stretching Handbook is a great resource for coaches and athletes. It offers a quick and easy reference to stretches for all areas of the body. It's size is an added bonus, making it easy to fit into a bag or back pocket."

Jill McIntosh
Coach - Australian Netball Team

"A comprehensive, helpful and easy-to-read publication. Great for amateurs and professionals."

Frank Farina
Former Member - Australian Socceroo Squad
Player / Coach - Brisbane Strikers

"As a sportsman and now in my role offering improved health and preventative health care, I see this as a very practical tool for people of all walks of life. May it encourage all people to stretch to new heights of health and well being."

Brendan Long (B.Ed.)
General Manager - Camp Eden Health Retreat

Many thanks to:

- My wife Jenny, for her love, devotion and belief in me;
- My family, for their continuous support and encouragement;
- Steve Hermiston, for your experience and guidance;
- All those who contributed generous personal endorsements; &
- Especially my brother Matt, whose friendship I treasure.

First published; September 1997.
Revised and updated; December 1998.

Publisher: Walkerbout Health
            PO Box 3063
            Robina Town Centre
            Queensland 4230
            AUSTRALIA

Telephone: +61 (0) 7 5525 3543
Facsimile: +61 (0) 7 5525 3526

E-mail: admin@thestretchinghandbook.com
Web Site: www.thestretchinghandbook.com

ISBN: 0 646 31049 6

CONTENTS

INTRODUCTION

As someone who has been involved in all aspects of sport, including coaching, lecturing, administrating and participating, I am well aware of the need for reliable, up-to-date information on all aspects of health, fitness, sport and exercise.

For the last ten years I have been desperately seeking a comprehensive guide to stretching, a book that takes stretching seriously, with a detailed list and picture of every possible sports-related stretch a person can do. In my search I found many books where stretching got a mention, but nothing more than a page or two of vague generalisations and a few stick figures performing some very basic stretches. So, I decided to stop searching and start writing.

The Stretching Handbook is written as an easy to use, quick reference guide. You don't have to read it from cover to cover to take advantage of the information it contains. Carry it with you and refer to it often. This is a back-pocket handbook not a sit-on-the-shelf text book.

If you want information on stretches for the back look under that section. If you want to know what stretching can do for you, have a read through some of the benefits in chapter 4. Or if you want to know why your muscles are sore after exercises refer to the chapter on physiology.

Whether you are just starting to exercise for the first time or are a seasoned veteran of professional sport, whether the closest you have come to sport is watching your children play on a Saturday morning or whether you are the professional coach of a national team, *The Stretching Handbook* will benefit you.

CHAPTER 1

PHYSIOLOGY AND FITNESS

A revolution is occurring in the health and fitness industry as this book is being written. Old rules are being discarded and new rules are being made. Every day there are advances in the health and fitness industry. There is a multitude of new information about exercise and while most people are aware of the importance of being fit and healthy, much of this new information is confusing and conflicting. People need to be kept up to date concerning the basics of how the body works and what should be done to achieve and maintain peak health and fitness.

THE PHYSIOLOGY OF MUSCLES AND TENDONS

Muscles are made up of thousands of tiny cylindrical cells called muscle fibres. These muscle fibres run parallel to each other and some can be as long as 30 cm. Muscles are connected to the bones by tendons, which consist of dense connective tissue. They are extremely strong yet very pliable. It is the muscle fibres and tendons that we need to stretch to gain the maximum benefits of good flexibility, and decrease the likelihood of injury.

HOW MUSCLES REACT TO EXERCISE

Exercise is a disciplined form of physical activity designed to place stress on the body. When the body recovers from that stress it is better prepared and more capable of performing that particular physical activity in the future.

During exercise many demands are made on the working muscles. One of the first things to occur to muscles when they are stressed beyond a comfortable, or submaximal level, is that the individual muscle fibres become inflamed.

Due to the increased need for oxygen and nutrients the heart pumps large amounts of blood to the working muscles which causes them to swell. In the extreme, this puts pressure on the nerve endings and may result in pain.

When the stress of exercise on the working muscles is excessive a lot of damage can occur to the individual muscle fibres. This damage includes minute tears within the individual muscle fibres, called micro tears, and combined with swelling, can result in pain, a decrease in athletic performance and the possibility of serious injury.

During exercise the heart continually pumps blood to the working muscles. When the oxygen and nutrients in the blood have been used, the working muscles push the blood back to the heart. When the exercising muscles stop, so does the force that pushes the blood back to the heart, this results in blood pooling. This is when large amounts of blood accumulate in the muscles and results in a lot of pain due to the increased pressure placed on nerve endings.

Muscles also produce waste products such as lactic acid during strenuous exercise. Restricted blood flow prevents the drainage of these waste products from the muscles which can lead to pain and damage.

This all sounds like bad news but exercise is beneficial. Correct exercise will improve the body but if taken to extremes the results are unfavourable and instead of reaping the rewards of physical activity, the result will be sore, stiff muscles.

Too much or inappropriate exercise can have a disastrous effect on performance and can result in serious injury. In later chapters this will be explained in depth.

FITNESS AND FLEXIBILITY

An individual's physical fitness depends on a vast number of components, flexibility is only one of these. Although flexibility is a vital part of physical fitness it is important to see it as only one spoke in the fitness wheel. Other components include strength, power, speed, endurance, balance, co-ordination, agility and skill, etc.

Although particular sports require different levels of each fitness component it is essential to plan a regular exercise or training program that covers all the spokes in the fitness wheel.

Football, for example, relies heavily on strength and power, however the exclusion of skill drills and flexibility training could lead to serious injury and poor performance. Strength and flexibility are of prime concern to a gymnast but a sound training program would also improve power, speed and endurance.

The same is true for each individual, while some people seem to be naturally strong or flexible it would be foolish for such a person to completely ignore the other components of physical fitness. This is why such athletes as ironmen and triathletes are often referred to as being totally fit, because their sport demands an even distribution of the components that make up physical fitness.

Defining the appropriate balance is the key to your health and fitness success and may require the assistance of a qualified, professional trainer.

CHAPTER 2

FLEXIBILITY - AN OVERVIEW

This book contains key information on both general and specific stretching and the programs required to achieve it, with a view to improving flexibility and decreasing the likelihood of sports injury. It is important to understand the basics of flexibility, and also look at the consequences of neglecting your flexibility as part of your overall health and fitness.

THE DANGERS AND LIMITATIONS OF POOR FLEXIBILITY

Flexibility refers to the range of movement which exists around a particular joint, that is, how far we can reach, bend and turn. Poor flexibility creates many problems and can be so damaging it is difficult to understand why most people do not stretch regularly, as this is the best way to improve flexibility.

Tight, stiff muscles limit our normal range of movement. In some cases, lack of flexibility can be a contributing factor to back and neck pain, while a simple stretching routine could help prevent this. In the extreme, lack of flexibility can mean it is difficult, for example, to even bend down or look over our shoulder.

Tight, stiff muscles interfere with proper muscle action. If the muscles cannot contract and relax efficiently, decreased performance and a lack of muscle movement control will result. Short, tight muscles also cause a dramatic loss of strength and power during physical activity.

In a small percentage of cases tight, stiff muscles can even have an effect on blood circulation. Good blood circulation is vitally important so that the muscles are able to receive adequate amounts of oxygen and nutrients. This can result in increased muscle fatigue and ultimately, the ability to recover from strenuous exercise and the muscles' repair process is impeded.

Any one of these factors can greatly increase the chance of becoming injured. Together they present a package that includes muscular discomfort, loss of performance, an increased risk of injury and a greater likelihood of repeated injury.

HOW IS FLEXIBILITY RESTRICTED ?

The muscular system needs to be flexible to achieve peak performance and stretching is the most effective way of developing and retaining flexible muscles and tendons. However a number of other factors also contribute to a decrease in flexibility.

Flexibility, or range of movement, can be restricted by both internal and external factors. Internal factors such as, bones, ligaments, muscle bulk, muscle length, tendons and skin all restrict the amount of movement at any particular joint. As an example, the human leg cannot bend forward beyond a straight position because of the structure of the bones and ligaments that make up the knee joint.

External factors such as age, gender, temperature, restrictive clothing and of course any injury or disability will also have an effect on one's flexibility.

FLEXIBILITY AND THE AGEING PROCESS

It is no secret that with each passing year muscles and joints seem to become stiffer and tighter. This is part of the ageing process and is caused by a combination of physical degeneration and inactivity. Although you can't help getting older this doesn't mean that you should give up trying to improve your flexibility.

Age should not be a barrier to a fit and active lifestyle but certain precautions should be taken as we get older. You just need to work at it for longer, be a little more patient and be a lot more careful.

*Bob Anderson, author of 'Stretching', recommends that everyone include stretching as part of their health and fitness regime but also warns that any one over the age of 35 should pay special attention to their flexibility and incorporate specific stretching workouts into their exercise program.

The benefits of flexibility, how important it is to our general well-being and how it can enhance athletic performance is covered in chapter 4.

* The Flex Factor by Bob Anderson. From 'Runners World' Feb. 1989. Vol. 24. N 2. Pg. 38 - 41.

CHAPTER 3

A STRETCHING STORY

Once upon a time there was an eager, young athlete ready to take on the world. He trained hard, ate right, got lots of rest and did all the things a budding young athlete should do.

His speciality was the 10 km run and he wasn't too bad either. His personal best was 32 minutes and 4 seconds. That's pretty good for a seventeen year old kid. But he longed to break the 30 minute barrier, he'd tried everything but nothing seemed to work.

His training program was well structured and very professional. He was disciplined and rarely wavered from his set training program. He incorporated long runs, tempo runs, interval training, strength work in the gym, hill running, cross country running, deep water running and various other training methods to try and improve his personal best. He even bought a mountain bike to introduce cross training into his program.

He always ate right, took extra vitamins and minerals to supplement his diet and always made sure that he drank plenty of water. He made sure he was well rested and even got the occasional massage to help his legs recover.

I met our budding young athlete at a local 'fun-run' where he had a good race and achieved a time that most people would be happy with. Although it was close to his personal best, it was still nowhere near his goal of breaking 30 minutes.

We got to talking and I could tell he was disheartened and frustrated. He explained to me that he had tried everything and nothing he did seemed to improve his personal best. I asked if he would mind if I attended one of his training sessions and he welcomed the idea of getting some fresh advice.

As it turned out, the next session that I could get to was an interval session at the local 400 metre track. As I arrived he was just finishing his warm-up with a few 'run throughs.' For this session he was going to do 8 x 400 metre intervals with plenty of rest in between each one.

As soon as he started the first interval I could tell what was wrong. His hamstrings and calf muscles were so tight that they restricted the normal range of movement of his legs to the extent that they shortened his stride length. For a tall guy with long legs his stride length was atrociously short.

After he finished his cool-down I asked him if he ever did any stretching. He replied quite honestly by saying he did none at all. Just to be sure we did a few flexibility tests for his back, hamstrings and calves. From these it was quite obvious that his flexibility was the major limiting factor in achieving his goal.

I went on to explain how his lack of flexibility was contributing to a shortened stride length, which in turn was making it difficult to improve his personal best time. Armed with this new bit of hope he eagerly wanted advice on how to incorporate stretching into his training program.

We sat down together and reviewed his training program for the next two weeks. We decided not to make any changes to the program itself, but simply add a general stretching workout to each session. The only advice I gave him was to add 10 minutes of stretching before each session, add another 15 minutes of stretching after each session and atleast 30 minutes of stretching each night.

The results didn't happen overnight, but within two weeks his general flexibility improved considerably. We then incorporated a number of specific stretches to further increase the flexibility of his hamstrings, calves and back.

The improvements over the next couple of months were remarkable. Not only did his times improve but his running style and technique also improved considerably.

The last time I spoke with our budding young athlete he still hadn't achieved his 30 minute goal, but his 400 metre time had dropped to just under 60 seconds. His 5 km personal best was right on 15 minutes and his 10 km personal best was now just under 31 minutes. I'm positive it is only a matter of time before he achieves his goal of breaking 30 minutes for 10 km.

Remembering that, except for adding stretching to his program, nothing else changed. We didn't add anything to his program and we didn't take anything away. All we did was incorporate basic stretching exercises as a regular part of his training and the results were remarkable.

Don't make the mistake of thinking that something as simple as stretching won't be effective. Stretching is a vital part of any exercise program and should be looked upon as being as important as any other part of your health and fitness.

CHAPTER 4

STRETCHING - THE BENEFITS

Stretching is the process of placing particular parts of the body in a position which will lengthen the muscles and tendons. Stretching is a simple and effective activity which helps to enhance athletic performance, decrease the likelihood of injury and minimise muscle soreness.

Upon undertaking a regular stretching program a number of changes occur within the body. Firstly, by placing particular parts of the body in certain positions, we are able to increase the length of muscles and tendons. As a result of this, a reduction in general muscle tension is achieved and our normal range of movement is increased.

By increasing our range of movement we are increasing the distance our limbs can move before damage occurs to the muscles and tendons. For example, the muscles and tendons in the back of our legs are put under great strain when kicking a football. Therefore, the more flexible and pliable those muscles are, the further our leg can travel forward before a strain or injury occurs to them.

The benefits of an extended range of movement includes: increased comfort; a greater ability to move freely; and a lessening of our susceptibility to injury.

There is a dangerous stretching myth that says, 'if you stretch too much you will lose both joint stability and muscle power'. This is totally untrue. By increasing our muscle and tendon length we are increasing the distance over which our muscles are able to contract. This results in a potential increase to our muscles' power and therefore increases our athletic ability, while also leading to an improvement in dynamic balance, or the ability to control our muscles.

We have all experienced what happens when you go for a run or to the gym for the first time in a few months. The following day our muscles are tight, sore, stiff and it's usually hard to even walk down a flight of stairs. This soreness that usually accompanies strenuous physical activity is often referred to as post exercise muscle soreness. This soreness is the result of micro tears, (minute tears within the muscle fibres), blood pooling and accumulated waste products, such as lactic acid. Stretching, as part of an effective cool-down, helps to alleviate this soreness by lengthening the individual muscle fibres, increasing blood circulation and removing waste products.

Fatigue is a major problem for everyone, especially those who exercise. It results in a decrease in both physical and mental performance. Increased flexibility through stretching can help prevent the effects of fatigue by taking pressure off the working muscles. Let me explain how this is so. For every muscle in the body there is an opposite or opposing muscle. If the opposing muscles are more flexible, the working muscles do not have to exert as much force against the opposing muscles. Therefore each movement of the working muscles actually takes less effort.

In summary, any person who experiences the benefits of stretching and increased flexibility is certainly more likely to feel good about themselves. This leads to a confidence and assuredness which helps to enhance physical performance and motivate the individual to participate in exercise.

CHAPTER 5

STRETCHING - THE FOUR TYPES

Stretching is slightly more technical than swinging your leg over a park bench. There are rules and methods which will maximise the benefits while minimising the risk of injury.

In this chapter we will be looking at the different types of stretching, the particular benefits, risks and uses, plus a description of how each type is performed.

The four types of stretching are:

1. *STATIC STRETCHING*
2. *PARTNER / OBJECT STRETCHING*
3. *PNF STRETCHING*
4. *DYNAMIC STRETCHING*

Each type of stretching has particular benefits for different sports and different individuals. I recommend that you start with static stretching and partner / object stretching. For improved flexibility incorporate PNF stretching into your program and only attempt dynamic stretching under the supervision of a professional sports coach.

IMPORTANT:
OBSERVE STRETCHING
RULES IN CHAPTER 6

1. Static Stretching

- very safe and effective
- limited threat of injury
- good for overall flexibility
- good for beginners and sedentary individuals

Static stretching is performed by placing the body into a position whereby the muscle (or group of muscles) to be stretched is under tension. Both the opposing muscle group (the muscles behind or in front of the stretched muscle), and the muscles to be stretched are relaxed. Then slowly and cautiously the body is moved to increase the tension of the muscle (or group of muscles) to be stretched. At this point the position is held or maintained to allow the muscles and tendons to lengthen. No outside external force is applied to the body, only forces generated by the opposing muscles.

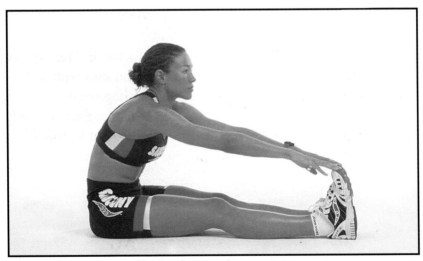

Fig 5.1 is a classic example of a static stretch, in which both the opposing muscles and the hamstring and back muscles are relaxed.

2. *PARTNER / OBJECT STRETCHING*

- helps to attain a greater range of movement
- slightly increased risk of injury
- beneficial for a deeper, more extensive stretch
- good for use on specific problem areas
- imperative for enhanced athletic performance
- very beneficial as part of a cool-down

This form of stretching is very similar to static stretching, however, another person or object is used to help further stretch the muscles. Due to the greater force applied to the muscles, this form of stretching is slightly more hazardous. Therefore it is very important that any object used is both solid and immovable. When using a partner it is imperative that no jerky or bouncing force is applied to the stretched muscle. So, choose your partner carefully, they must be responsible for your safety while stretching.

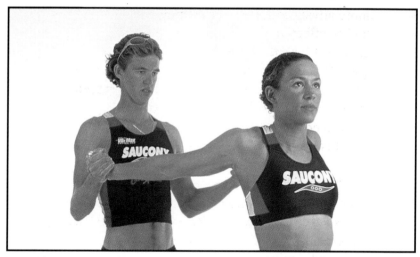

Fig 5.2 is an example of using a partner to stretch the chest and shoulder muscles.

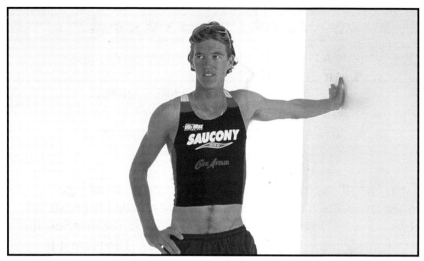

Fig 5.3 shows a different way to get a similar stretch using an object. Notice that both of these stretches are more effective when a partner or object is used.

3.   *PNF Stretching*
(Proprioceptive Neuromuscular Facilitation)

- more advanced form of stretching
- highly effective
- excellent for specific muscle groups
- good for rehabilitation
- promotes both flexibility and muscular strength
- increased risk of injury
- needs a conditioning phase before maximum effort is used

The area to be stretched is positioned so that the muscle is under tension. The athlete then contracts the stretched muscle group for 5 - 6 seconds while a partner applies sufficient resistance to inhibit movement. The effort of contraction should be relevant to the level of conditioning. The contracted muscle group is then relaxed and a controlled stretch is applied for about 30 seconds.

The athlete is then allowed 30 seconds to recover and the process is repeated 2 - 4 times.

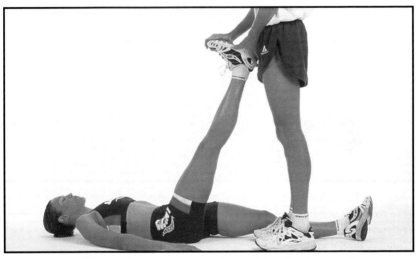

Fig 5.4 The athlete and partner assume the position for the stretch.

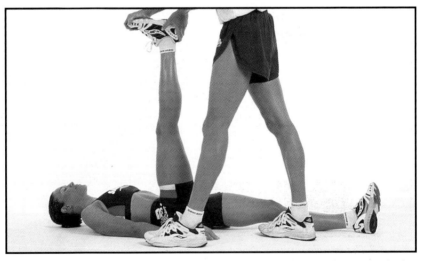

Fig 5.5 The partner then extends the body limb until the muscle is stretched and tension is felt.

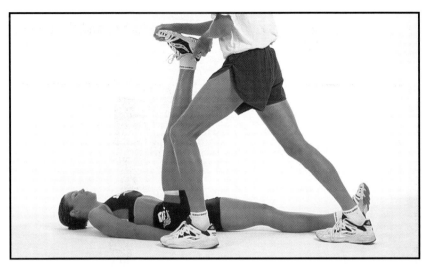

*Fig 5.6 The athlete then contracts the stretched muscle for 5 - 6 seconds and the partner **must** inhibit all movement. (The force of the contraction should be relevant to the condition of the muscle. For example, if the muscle has been injured, do not apply a maximum contraction).*

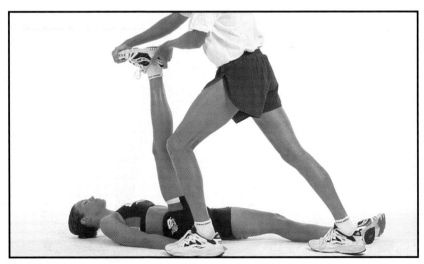

Fig 5.7 The muscle group is then relaxed, then immediately and cautiously pushed past its normal range of movement for about 30 seconds. Allow 30 seconds recovery before repeating the procedure 2 - 4 times.

4. DYNAMIC STRETCHING

- only used by professional, well trained, highly conditioned athletes
- only for specific sports
- high risk of injury (use under the supervision of a professional sports coach)
- more for conditioning than flexibility
- should only be used after a high level of flexibility has been established

A controlled, soft bounce or swinging motion is used to force a particular body part past its usual range of movement. The force of the bounce or swing is gradually increased but should never become radical or uncontrolled.

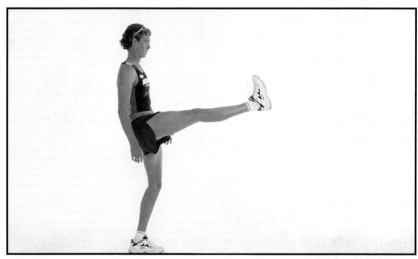

Fig 5.8 is an example of a dynamic stretch for the hamstring muscles. This stretch is especially useful for people involved in sports requiring kicking.
Remember: *Take note of the above points and only use under the supervision of a professional sports coach.*

CHAPTER 6

STRETCHING - THE RULES

As with most activities there are rules and guidelines to ensure that they are safe. Stretching is no exception. Stretching can be extremely dangerous and harmful if done incorrectly. It is vitally important that the following rules be adhered to, both for safety and for maximising the potential benefits of stretching.

The six rules are:

> 1. *WARM-UP PRIOR TO STRETCHING*
> 2. *STRETCH BEFORE AND AFTER EXERCISE*
> 3. *STRETCH ALL MAJOR MUSCLES AND THEIR OPPOSING MUSCLE GROUPS*
> 4. *STRETCH GENTLY AND SLOWLY (AVOID BOUNCING UNLESS SUPERVISED BY A PROFESSIONAL SPORTS COACH)*
> 5. *STRETCH ONLY TO THE POINT OF TENSION*
> 6. *BREATHE SLOWLY AND EASILY*

Now let's take a close look at why each of these rules are important.

1. WARM-UP PRIOR TO STRETCHING

This first rule is often overlooked and can lead to serious injury if broken. Trying to stretch muscles which have not been warmed, is like trying to stretch old, dry rubber bands, they may snap.

Warming up prior to stretching does a number of beneficial things, but primarily its purpose is to prepare the body and mind for more strenuous activity. One of the ways it achieves this is by helping to increase the body's core temperature while also increasing the body's muscle temperature. By increasing muscle temperature we are helping to make the muscles loose, supple and pliable. This is essential to ensure the maximum benefit is gained from your stretching.

The correct warm-up, also has the effect of increasing both your heart rate and your respiratory rate. This increases blood flow which in turn increases the delivery of oxygen and nutrients to the working muscles. All this helps to prepare the muscles and tendons for stretching.

A correct warm-up should consist of a light physical activity. Both the intensity and duration of the warm-up (or how hard and how long), should be governed by the fitness level of the participating athlete, although a correct warm-up for most people should take about ten minutes and result in a light sweat. Remember, warm muscles are flexible muscles, while cold muscles may snap like an old, dry rubber band.

2. STRETCH BEFORE AND AFTER EXERCISE

The question often arises, "should I stretch before or after exercise ?" This is not an either or situation, both are essential. It is no good stretching after exercise and counting that as your pre-exercise stretch for next time. Stretching after exercise has a totally different purpose to stretching before exercise. The two are not the same.

The purpose of stretching before exercise, is to help prevent injury. Stretching does this by lengthening the muscles and tendons, which in turn increases your range of movement. This ensures that you are able to move freely without restriction or injury occurring.

However, stretching after exercise has a very different role. Its purpose is primarily to aid in the repair and recovery of the muscles and tendons. By lengthening the muscles and tendons, stretching helps to prevent tight muscles and delayed muscle soreness which usually accompanies strenuous exercise.

After exercise your stretching should be done as part of a cool-down. The cool-down will vary depending on the duration and intensity of exercise undertaken, but will usually consist of five to ten minutes of very light physical activity and be followed by five to ten minutes of general stretching.

An effective cool-down involving light physical activity and stretching will help to: rid waste products from the muscles; prevent blood pooling; and promote the delivery of oxygen and nutrients to the muscles. All this assists in returning the body to a pre-exercise level, thus aiding the recovery process.

3. STRETCH ALL MAJOR MUSCLES AND THEIR OPPOSING MUSCLE GROUPS

When stretching, it is vitally important that you pay attention to all the major muscle groups in the body. Just because your particular sport may place a lot of emphasis on the legs, for example, it does not mean that you can neglect the muscles of your upper body in your stretching routine.

All the muscles play an important part in any physical activity, not just a select few. Muscles in the upper body, for example, are extremely important in any running sport, they play a vital role in the stability and balance of the body during the running motion. Therefore it is important to keep them both flexible and supple.

Every muscle in the body has an opposing muscle which acts against it. For example, the muscles in the front of the leg, (the quadriceps) are opposed by the muscles in the back of the leg, (the hamstrings). These two groups of muscles provide a resistance to each other to balance the body. If one of these groups of muscles becomes stronger or more flexible than the opposing group, it is likely to lead to imbalances which can result in injury or postural problems. For example, hamstring tears are a common injury in most running sports. They are often caused by strong quadriceps and weak, inflexible hamstrings. This imbalance puts a great deal of pressure on the hamstrings and usually results in a muscle tear or strain.

4. STRETCH GENTLY AND SLOWLY, (AVOID BOUNCING UNLESS SUPERVISED BY A PROFESSIONAL SPORTS COACH)

Following this rule will help you attain the maximum possible benefits from your stretching. Stretching slowly and gently helps to relax your muscles, which in turn makes stretching more pleasurable and beneficial. This will also help to avoid muscle tears and strains which can be caused by rapid, jerky movements.

5. STRETCH ONLY TO THE POINT OF TENSION

Stretching is not an activity which was meant to be painful, it should be pleasurable, relaxing and very beneficial, although many people believe that to get the most from their stretching they need to be in constant pain. This is one of the greatest mistakes people make when stretching. Let me explain why.

When the muscles and tendons are stretched to the point of pain, the body employs a defence mechanism called the 'stretch reflex'. This is the body's safety measure to prevent serious damage occurring to the muscles and tendons. The 'stretch reflex' protects the muscles and tendons by contracting them, thereby preventing them from being stretched.

To avoid the 'stretch reflex', avoid pain. Never push yourself beyond what is comfortable. Only stretch to the point where tension is felt in the muscles. To get the greatest benefits, remember the fourth rule, stretch gently and slowly and avoid bouncing unless supervised by a professional sports coach.

6. BREATHE SLOWLY AND EASILY

Many people unconsciously hold their breath while stretching. This causes tension in the muscles which in turn makes it very difficult to stretch. To avoid this, remember to breathe slowly and easily during your stretching. This promotes blood flow and increases the delivery of oxygen and nutrients to the muscles. Breathing slowly and easily also helps to relax the muscles which makes stretching easier and more beneficial.

The purpose of these rules is twofold. Firstly, to ensure that your stretching is safe and injury free, and secondly to ensure that you gain the greatest possible benefits from your stretching.

Just imagine how good you will feel when you take your stretching seriously: warming up before stretching; stretching before and after you exercise; stretching all major muscles and their opposing muscle groups; stretching gently and slowly; and, only stretching to the point of tension while breathing slowly and easily.

CHAPTER 7

STRETCHING - THE HOW TO'S

This chapter holds crucial information concerning the particular how to's, or basic mechanics of stretching.

WHEN TO STRETCH ?

As we have discussed earlier it is important to stretch both before and after exercise. But when else should you stretch?

Why not stretch periodically throughout the entire day? It's a great way to keep loose and to help ease the stress of everyday life.

One of the most productive ways to utilise your time is to stretch while you are watching television. Start with five minutes of marching or jogging on the spot then take a seat on the floor in front of the television and kill two birds with one stone.

Your stretching needs to be as important as the rest of your training. If you are involved in any competitive type of sport or exercise then it is crucial that you make time for specific stretching workouts. Set time aside to work on particular areas that are tight or stiff. The more involved and committed you are to your exercise and fitness the more time and effort you will need to commit to stretching.

Competition is a time when great demands are placed on the body, therefore it is vitally important that you are in peak physical condition. Your flexibility should be at its best just before competition. Too many injuries are caused by the sudden exertion which is needed for any sort of competitive sport. Get strict on your stretching before competition.

FREQUENCY AND DURATION

How long should I hold each stretch? How long should I stretch for? How often should I stretch?

These are the most commonly asked questions when discussing the topic of stretching. Although there are conflicting responses to these questions, through a study of research literature and personal experience, I believe what follows is currently the most correct and beneficial information.

The question which causes the most conflict is, how long should I hold each stretch for? Some text will tell you that as little as ten seconds is enough. This is a bare minimum. Ten seconds is only just enough time for the muscles to relax and start to lengthen. For any real benefit to your flexibility you must hold each stretch for at least thirty seconds and for maximum benefit the recommendation is up to sixty seconds.

The time you commit to your stretching will be relative to your level of involvement in your particular sport. So, for people looking to increase their general level of health and fitness, a minimum of about twenty seconds will be enough. However, if you are involved in high level competitive sport you need to hold each stretch for at least forty seconds and start to extend that to sixty seconds and beyond.

This same principal of adjusting your level of commitment to your level of involvement in your sport applies to the number of times you should stretch each muscle group. For example, the beginner should stretch each muscle group two to three times. However, if you are involved at a more advanced level in your sport you should stretch each muscle group three to five times.

How long should you stretch for? The same principal applies. For the beginner, about ten to fifteen minutes is enough. For the professional athlete, anything up to two hours. If you feel you are somewhere between the beginner and the professional adjust the time you spend stretching accordingly.

Please don't be impatient with your stretching. You don't get fit in a couple of weeks, so don't expect miracles with your stretching. Looking long term, some muscles and tendons may need a minimum of three months of intense stretching to see any real improvement. So stick with it, it is well worth the effort.

SEQUENCING OF YOUR PROGRAM

When starting a stretching program it is a good idea to start with a general range of stretches for the entire body, instead of just a select few. The idea of this is to reduce overall muscle tension and to increase the mobility of your joints and limbs.

The next step should be to increase overall flexibility by starting to extend the muscles and tendons beyond their normal range of movement. Following this, work on specific areas that are tight or important for your particular sport. Remember, all this takes time. This sequence of stretches may take up to three months for you to see real improvement, especially if you have no background in agility based activities or are heavily muscled.

No data exists on what order you should do your stretches in. However, it is recommended that you start with sitting stretches, because there is less chance of injury while sitting, before moving on to standing stretches. To make it easier you may want to start with the ankles and move up to the neck or vice versa. It really doesn't matter as long as you cover all the major muscle groups and their opposing muscles.

POSTURE WHILE STRETCHING

Posture while stretching is one of the most neglected aspects of stretching. It is important to be aware of how crucial it can be to the overall benefits of your stretching. Bad posture and incorrect technique can cause imbalances in the muscles which can lead to injury.

In many instances a major muscle group can be made up of a number of different muscles. If your posture is sloppy or incorrect your stretching may put more emphasis on one particular muscle in that muscle group, thus causing an imbalance which could lead to injury.

For example, when stretching the hamstrings (the muscles at the back of the legs) it is imperative that you keep both feet pointing up. If your feet fall to the side this will put undue stress on one particular part of the hamstrings which will result in a muscle imbalance.

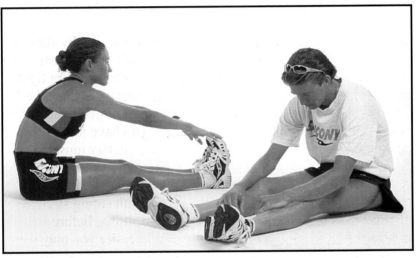

Fig 7.1 shows the difference between good posture and bad posture. Note the athlete on the left, feet upright and back straight. The athlete on the right is at greater risk of causing a muscular imbalance which may lead to injury.

The stretches shown at the back of this book all demonstrate correct posture, so please follow and copy them perfectly, do not change or modify them in any way.

CHAPTER 8

STRETCHING - THE INJURY PREVENTER

Sports Medicine Australia states that 1 out of every 17 partici-pants of sport and exercise will suffer an injury of some kind while engaged in their chosen sport. This is even higher for contact sports like Rugby League. But equally staggering is the fact that many of these injuries may have been prevented.

While preventative measures such as warming up, obeying the rules, using protective equipment and plain common-sense are all useful, stretching can play a vital role in helping to prevent the occurrence of injury. Unfortunately stretching is one area of athletic preparation often neglected.

Do not underestimate its benefits. Don't make the mistake of thinking that something as simple as stretching won't be effective. Stretching is a vital part of any exercise program and should be looked upon as being as important as any other part of your health and fitness.

HOW DOES STRETCHING PREVENT INJURY ?

One of the greatest benefits of stretching is that we are able to increase the length of our muscles and tendons. This leads to an increased range of movement, which means that our limbs and joints can move further before an injury occurs. For example, if the muscles of our neck are tight and inflexible this limits our ability to look behind us. If for some reason our head is turned backwards, past our normal range of movement, in a football scrum for example, this could result in a muscle tear or strain. We can help to prevent this from happening by increasing the flexibility, and the range of movement, of our neck muscles.

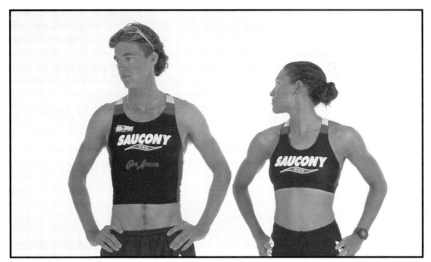

Fig 8.1 The athlete on the left has poor neck flexibility. This person is under an increased risk of injuring his neck if forced to turn his head quickly. The athlete on the right has good neck flexibility.

Obviously, while injuries can occur at any time, they are more likely to occur if the muscles are fatigued, tight and depleted of energy. Fatigued, tight muscles are also less capable of performing the skills required for each particular sport. Stretching can help prevent injury by promoting recovery and decreasing soreness. Stretching ensures that our muscles and tendons are in good working order.

While stretching is extremely effective, other techniques are also beneficial for aiding in the recovery process and thus helping to prevent injury. A very beneficial practice for both athletes and people who live a sedentary lifestyle is to lie on your back with your buttocks against a wall and your legs suspended vertically up the wall. This helps to drain waste products from the legs and also results in de-oxygenated blood being forced back to the heart where it can be re-oxygenated and distributed around the body. This is also a very good practice for people who have swollen feet and legs from standing for long periods of time.

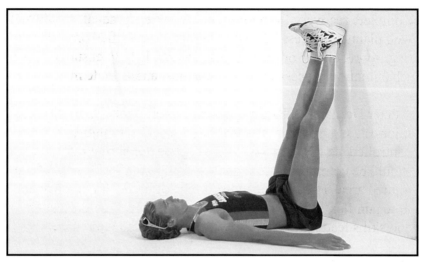

Fig 8.2 This practice is extremely beneficial for athletes as well as people who live a sedentary lifestyle.

INJURY REHABILITATION

Obviously, it is better to prevent an injury than to manage one. While stretching plays an important part in any rehabilitation process it is not the first course of action. Rather, in the event of an injury, it is important initially that you apply correct first aid principles immediately.

If a muscle strain or tear occurs, you should apply what is known as the R.I.C.E.R. regime for at least 48 to 72 hours. This involves the application of **Rest**, **Ice**, **Compression**, **Elevation** and obtaining a **Referral** for appropriate medical treatment. Where the R.I.C.E.R. regime has been used immediately after the occurrence of an injury, it has been shown to significantly improve recovery time. R.I.C.E.R. forms the first and perhaps most important stage of injury rehabilitation, providing the early base for the recovery of injury. (For more detailed information on the R.I.C.E.R. regime please consult a sports first aid handbook.)

Complete recovery from injury needs to be a gradual, steady and well planned process. Consultation with a qualified professional (e.g. sports doctor or physiotherapist) can help to ensure that the rehabilitation process occurs in the most appropriate manner.

* Peter Dornan and Richard Dunn, in their book 'Sporting Injuries', suggest that after the initial reaction to injury is controlled, as with the R.I.C.E.R. regime, rehabilitation exercises should be commenced to regain all components of fitness of the injured area. The specific aims of rehabilitation at this stage are to regain flexibility, strength, endurance, power, co-ordination and skills leading to the normal function of the injured area.

Dornan and Dunn go on to say that it is important that stretching exercises be initiated early if normal flexibility is to be regained and it is especially important to regain flexibility, not only of the injured area, but also of the muscles and tendons around the injured area.

Remember that short or tight muscles are more at risk of injury. You must therefore continue to pay attention to the flexibility of your injured area, even after full recovery, to ensure that you do not re-injure yourself.

* Sporting Injuries; P. Dornan & R. Dunn. Published by University of Queensland Press, 1987.

CHAPTER 9

FLEXIBILITY TESTING

To really take advantage of the many benefits of stretching you should consider keeping a record of your flexibility. For sports trainers and coaches, in particular, it is vitally important that you test and chart your serious athletes' flexibility on a regular basis. This is important for two reasons.

Firstly, it provides a starting point from which to measure improvements and gives an indication of any areas which may be weak or inflexible.

Secondly, in the event of an injury, this baseline flexibility provides a goal to achieve before resuming exercise or returning to competition. As discussed in the previous chapter, it is important that you regain your flexibility after an injury. Therefore having a record of what your flexibility was before the injury is very useful as a target to achieve.

During the year set a minimum standard of flexibility for the activities you are engaged in. If you become injured, it should be your goal to achieve the minimum standard of flexibility required for that activity before returning to exercise, competition or strenuous training.

What follows is a brief example of a few basic flexibility tests. These are probably the most commonly used tests but they are by no means the only ones. If you require more, consult a professional sports trainer for ideas about tests that are particular to your sport. Remember the stretching rules in chapter 6 and once a test is used it is important not to vary it in any way. It must be kept the same each time it is used.

All the following tests are best done using a goniometer, a devise for measuring body limb angles. If you do not have access to a goniometer any standard 360 degree protractor will give you a good indication of the angle at a particular joint.

SIT AND REACH TEST

The sit and reach test is probably the most common test used to measure flexibility in the back, hip and hamstring muscles.

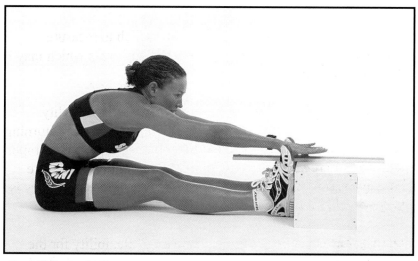

Fig 9.1 Sit on the floor with your legs straight and your feet flat against an upright board. Bend forward reaching towards, or as far past, your toes as possible. This test will give you a good indication of your hamstring, hip and back flexibility. Record the distance reached.

SHOULDER FLEXIBILITY TEST

Unfortunately, participants in sports such as, swimming, tennis (or any racket sport), any of the throwing events in athletics and especially contact sports, are extremely susceptible to injuries of the shoulder. Shoulder flexibility should be a prime concern for anyone participating in these sports.

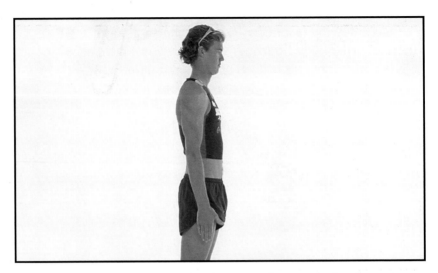

Fig 9.2 Stand upright with your hand pointing down, as in the above picture. In this position the hand represents the 0 degree position.

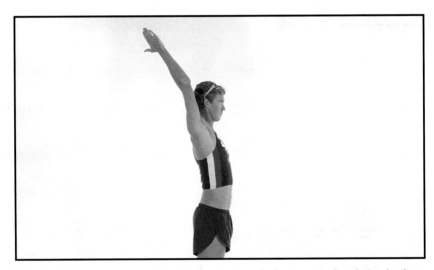

Fig 9.3 Raise your arm directly forward and above your head. Its furthest point is then recorded. An average acceptable reading of 180 degrees is expected for athletes.

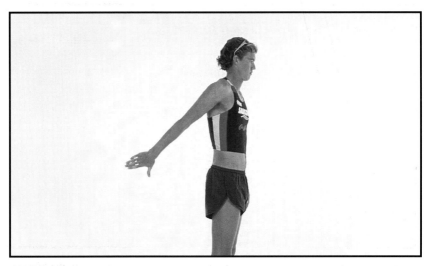

Fig 9.4 Now move your arm down and behind your back to its furthest position. This measurement is recorded and should exceed 50 degrees.

HAMSTRING FLEXIBILITY TEST

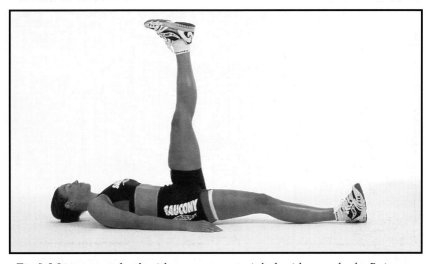

Fig 9.5 Lie on your back with your arms straight beside your body. Raise your leg as far up as possible. Keep your leg straight. Measure the angle at the hip joint. An angle of 90 degrees is considered average to good.

CHAPTER 10

THE STRETCHES

What follows is a detailed description of nearly 100 different stretches. These are not specific to any particular sport or any particular person. Of course all of them will not be relevant to everyone, however, I am sure that you will find a great number of them suitable for what you require.

Each stretch will be accompanied by a picture and a description of how it is to be performed. Every stretch has also been given a rating.

- Stretches rated *'GENERAL'* are safe for everybody.
- Stretches rated *'INTERMEDIATE'* are for people who are physically active.
- Stretches rated *'ADVANCED'* are only for well conditioned professional athletes.

You will also note that the stretches have been arranged to correspond with particular body parts. For example, if you are looking for stretches for the shoulders look under that particular heading. The stretches have been arranged so as to start with the neck and work down to the ankles. There is also an index on the following page to assist in finding individual stretches.

Important note; remember to follow the ratings outlined above and the stretching rules in chapter 6. If you have any pre-existing injuries or ailments please consult a sports doctor or physiotherapist before attempting any of the stretches.

INDEX OF STRETCHES

1.   NECK

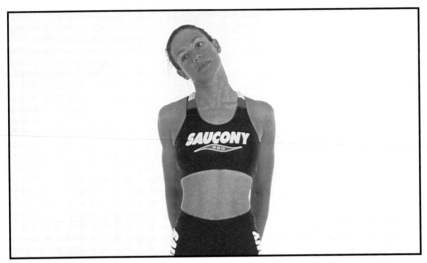

Fig 10.1 Look forward. Keep your head up. Slowly move your ear towards your shoulder. It is important to keep your hands behind your back and do not lift your shoulder up to your ear.

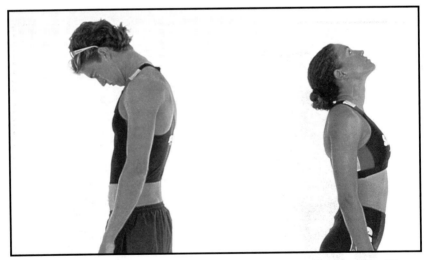

Fig 10.2 Stand upright. Let your chin fall forward towards your chest. Then lift your head, looking upwards as if trying to point up with your chin.

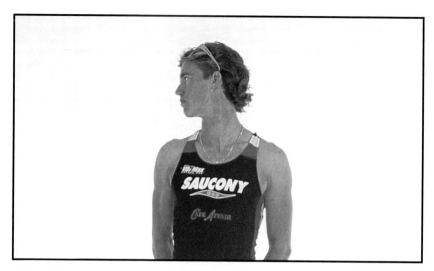

Fig 10.3 Stand upright. Keep your shoulders still and your head up. Slowly rotate your chin towards your shoulder.   ***GENERAL***

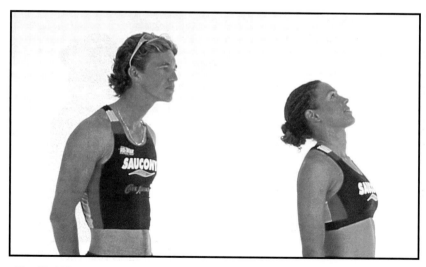

Fig 10.4 Keep your head up. Push your head forward by sticking your chin out. Then retract your head backwards.   ***GENERAL***

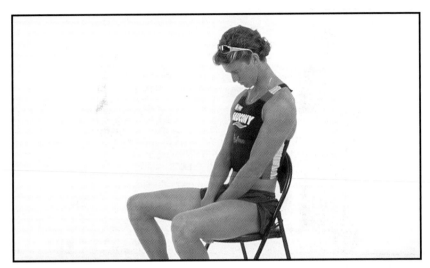

Fig 10.5 Sitting on a chair. Cross your arms over and hang on to the chair between your legs. Let your head fall forward. Lean backwards.

GENERAL

2   SHOULDERS

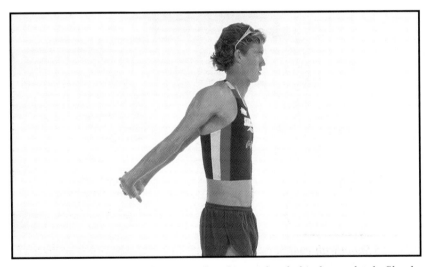

Fig 10.6 Stand upright. Clasp your hands together behind your back. Slowly lift your hands upward.

GENERAL

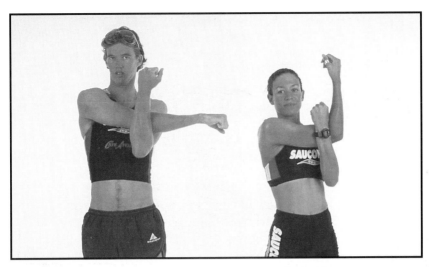

Fig 10.7 Stand upright. Place one arm across your body. Keep your arm parallel to the ground. Or for a slightly different stretch bend your arm at 90 degrees. Pull your elbow towards your opposite shoulder. **GENERAL**

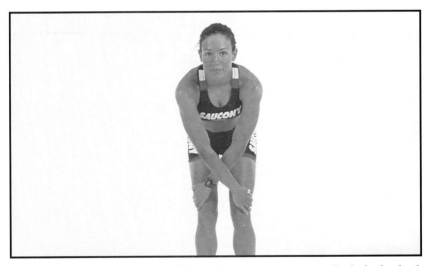

Fig 10.8 Stand with your knees bent. Cross your arms over. Grab the back of your knees. Start to raise upwards until you feel tension in your upper back and shoulders. **GENERAL**

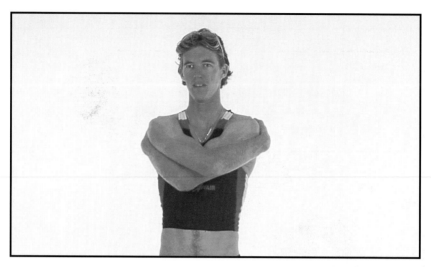

Fig 10.9 Stand upright. Wrap your arms around your shoulders as if hugging yourself. Pull your shoulders back. **GENERAL**

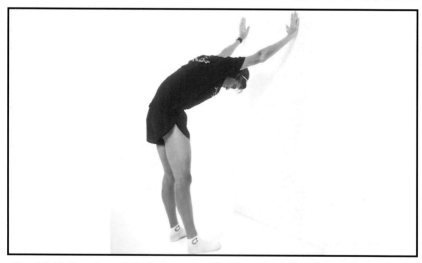

Fig 10.10 Stand upright facing a wall. Place both hands on the wall just above your head. Slowly lower your shoulders as if moving your chin towards the ground. **GENERAL**

3 ARMS

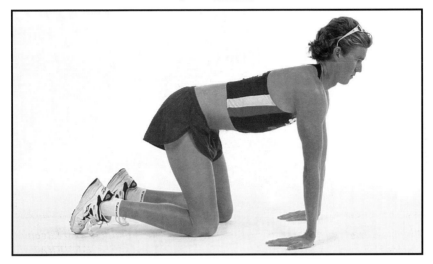

Fig 10.11 Crouching on your knees and hands with your forearms facing forward and hands pointing backwards. Slowly move rearward. (biceps and forearms). **GENERAL**

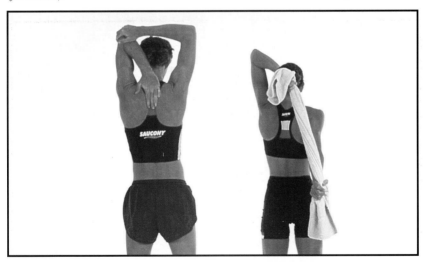

Fig 10.12 Stand with your hand behind your neck and your elbow pointing upwards. Use your other hand to pull your elbow down. Or hold onto a towel with both hands, using your lower arm to pull downwards. (triceps). **GENERAL**

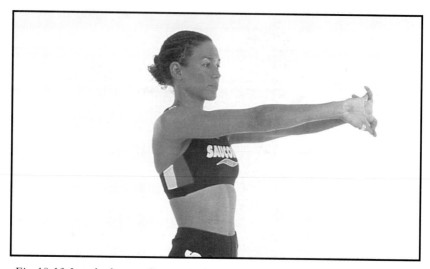

Fig 10.13 Interlock your fingers in front of your chest. Straighten your arms and turn the palms of your hands outwards. (forearms).   **GENERAL**

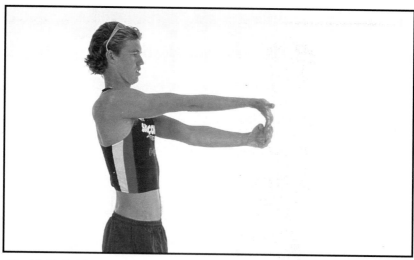

Fig 10.14 Hold onto your fingers. Turn your palms outwards. Straighten your arm. Pull your fingers back using your other hand. (forearms).

GENERAL

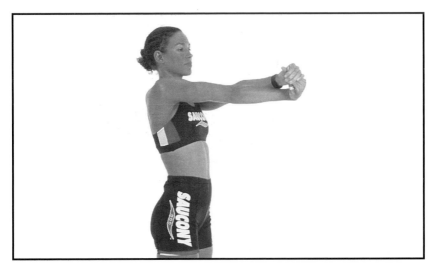

Fig 10.15 Place one arm straight out in front, parallel to the ground. Rotate your wrist down and outwards. Use your other hand to further rotate your hand upwards. (forearms).   GENERAL

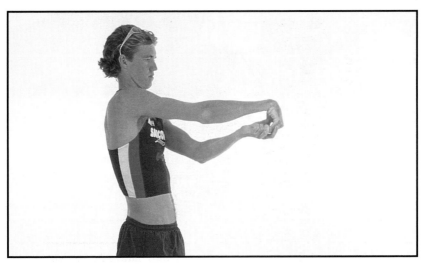

Fig 10.16 Hold on to your fingers. Straighten your arm. Pull your fingers towards your body. (wrists).   GENERAL

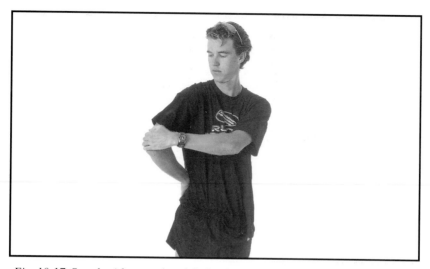

Fig 10.17 Stand with your hand behind the middle of your back and your elbow pointing out. Reach over with your other hand and gently pull your elbow forward. (rotators). **GENERAL**

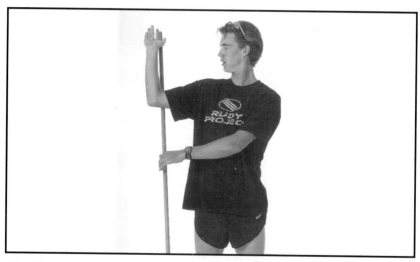

Fig 10.18 Stand with your arm out and your forearm pointing upwards at 90 degrees. Place a broom stick in your hand and behind your elbow. With your other hand pull the bottom of the broom stick forward. (rotators).

INTERMEDIATE

54

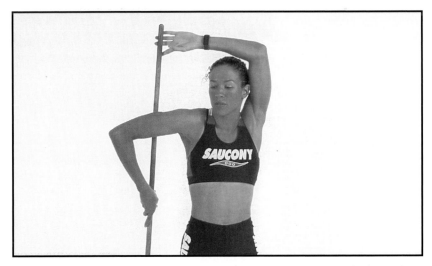

Fig 10.19 Stand with your arm out and your forearm pointing downwards at 90 degrees. Place a broom stick in your hand and behind your elbow. With your other hand pull the top of the broom stick forward. (rotators).

INTERMEDIATE

4.   CHEST

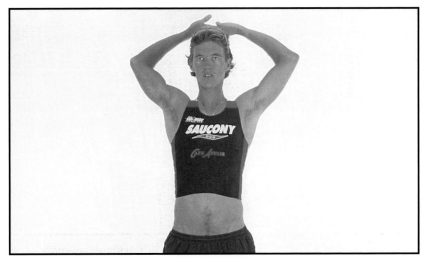

Fig 10.20 Stand upright. Interlock your fingers. Bend your arms and place them above your head. Force your elbows and hands backwards.

GENERAL

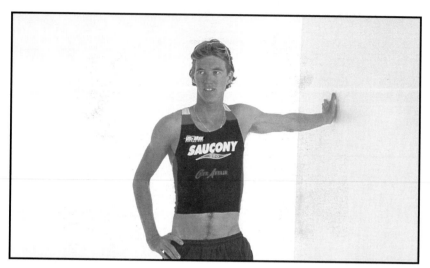

Fig 10.21 Stand with your arm extended to the rear and parallel to the ground. Hold on to an immovable object. Turn your shoulders and body away from your outstretched arm. **GENERAL**

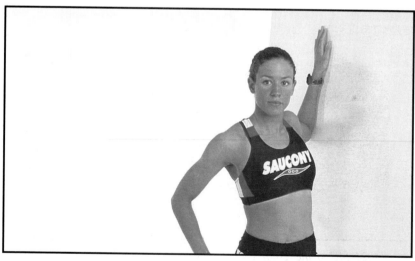

Fig 10.22 Stand with your arm extended and your forearm at right angles to the ground. Rest your forearm against an immovable object. Turn your shoulders and body away from your extended arm. **GENERAL**

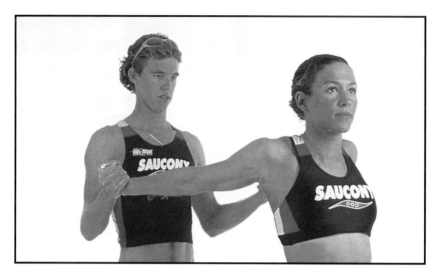

Fig 10.23 Extend both of your arms parallel to the ground. Have the partner hold on to your hands. Slowly pull your arms backwards. Remember to keep your arms parallel to the ground. **INTERMEDIATE**

5 BACK

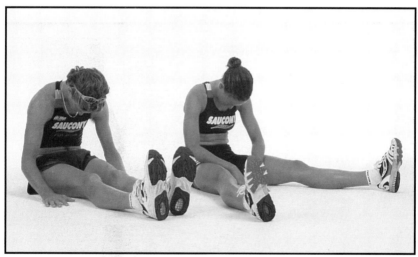

Fig 10.24 Sit on the ground with your legs straight out in front or at 45 degrees apart. Keep your toes pointing upwards. Rest your arms by your side or on your lap. Relax your back and neck. Let your head and chest fall forward. **GENERAL**

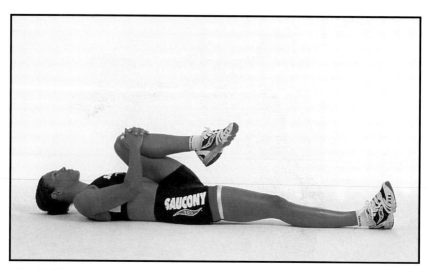

Fig 10.25 Lie on your back. Keep one leg flat on the ground. Bring your other knee up to your chest. **GENERAL**

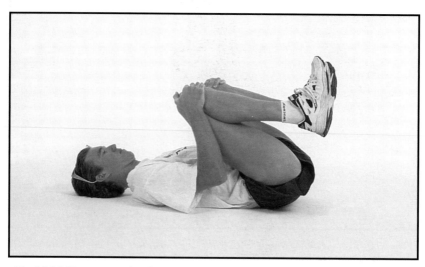

Fig 10.26 Lie on your back. Bring both knees up to your chest.

GENERAL

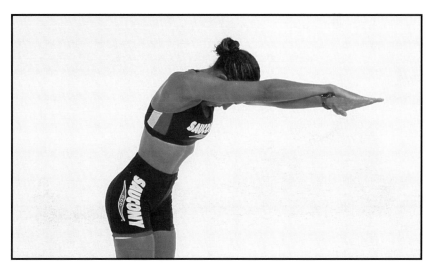

Fig 10.27 Stand with your arms crossed over. Push your hands forward as far as possible. Let your head fall forward. **GENERAL**

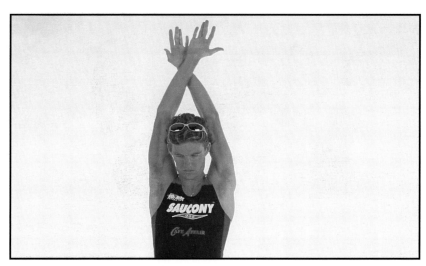

Fig 10.28 Stand with your arms crossed over. Raise them above your head. Reach up as far as you can. **GENERAL**

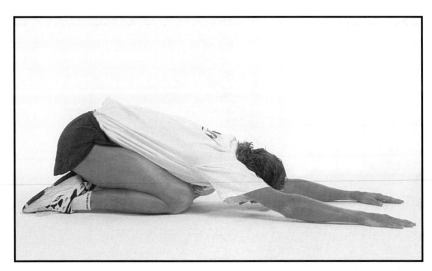

Fig 10.29 Kneel on the ground. Reach forward with your hands. Let your head fall forward. Push your buttocks towards your feet.   ***GENERAL***

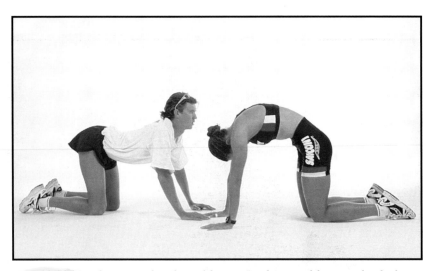

Fig 10.30 Kneel on your hands and knees. Look up and let your back slump downwards. Then let your head fall forward and arch your back upwards.
GENERAL

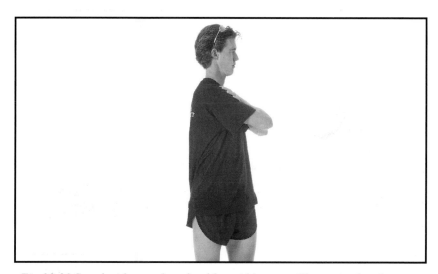

Fig 10.31 Stand with your feet shoulder width apart. Place your hands across your chest. Keeping your back and shoulders upright, slowly rotate your shoulders to one side. ***GENERAL***

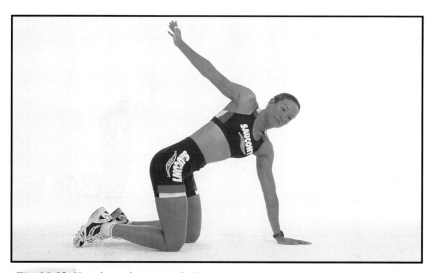

Fig 10.32 Kneel on the ground. Raise one arm. Rotate your shoulders and look upwards. Rotate your middle back. ***INTERMEDIATE***

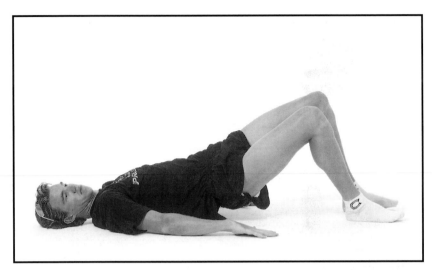

Fig 10.33 Lie on your back. Bring your feet towards your buttocks. Raise your stomach. Keep your hands by your side. Slowly rotate your hips from left to right. **INTERMEDIATE**

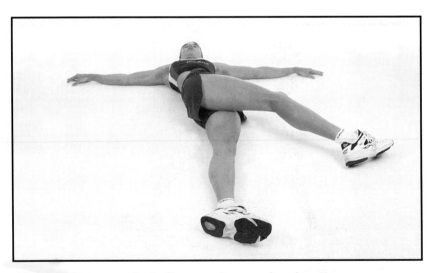

Fig 10.34 Lie on your back. Cross one leg over the other. Keep your arms out to the side and both legs straight. Let your back and hips rotate with your leg.
INTERMEDIATE

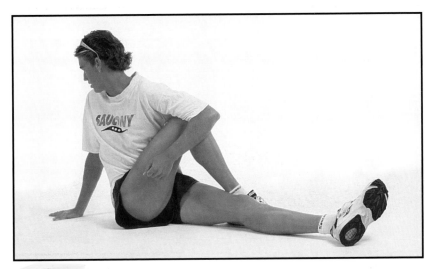

Fig 10.35 Sit with one leg straight and the other leg crossed over your knee. Turn your shoulders and put your arm against your raised knee to help rotate your shoulders and back.   ***INTERMEDIATE***

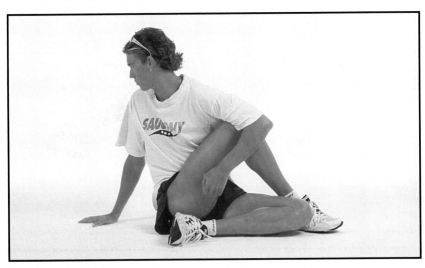

Fig 10.36 Sit with one leg bent and the other leg crossed over your knee. Turn your shoulders and put your arm against your raised knee to help rotate your shoulders and back.   ***INTERMEDIATE***

6. STOMACH

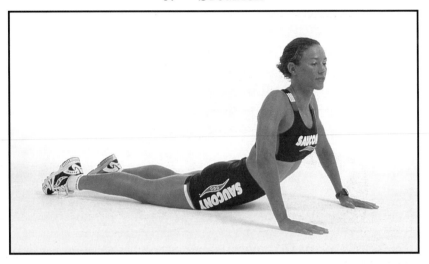

Fig 10.37 Lie face down. Bring your hands close to your shoulders. Keep your hips on the ground. Look forward. Raise up by straightening your arms.

GENERAL

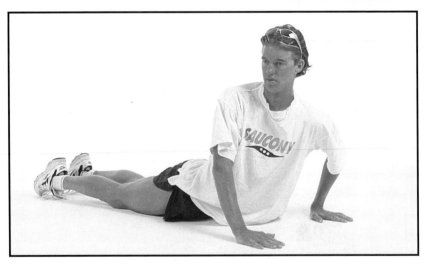

Fig 10.38 Lie face down. Bring your hands close to your shoulders. Keep your hips on the ground. Look forward. Raise up by straightening your arms. Slowly bend one arm and rotate that shoulder towards the ground.

INTERMEDIATE

7. SIDES

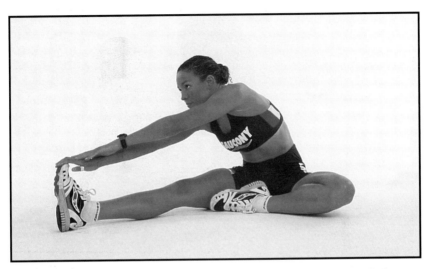

Fig 10.39 Sit with one leg straight out to the side and your toes pointing up. Bring your other foot up to your knee. Let your head fall forward. Reach towards the outside of your toes with both hands. **GENERAL**

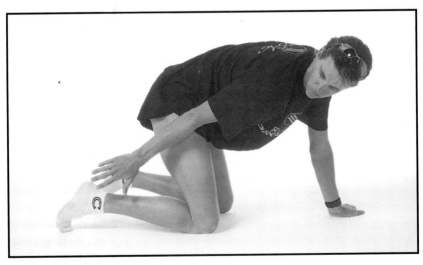

Fig 10.40 Kneel on your hands and knees. Take one hand and reach around towards your ankle. Keep your back parallel to the ground. **GENERAL**

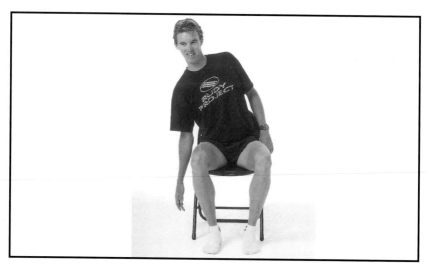

Fig 10.41 Sitting on a chair with your feet flat on the ground. Looking straight ahead and keeping your body upright. Slowly bend to the left or right, reaching towards the ground with one hand. Do not bend forward.

INTERMEDIATE

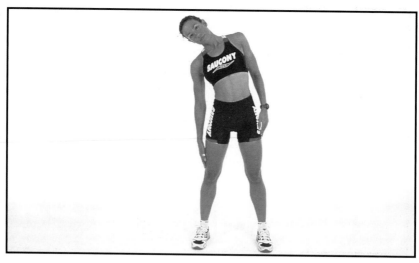

Fig 10.42 Stand with your feet about shoulder width apart. Look forward. Keep your body upright. Slowly bend to the left or right. Reach down your leg with your hand. Do not bend forward. **INTERMEDIATE**

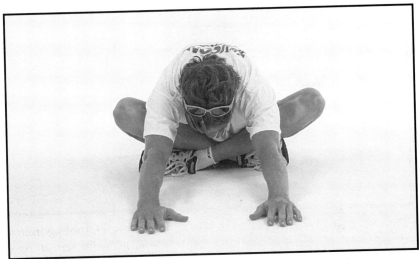

Fig 10.43 Sit cross legged. Keep your back straight. Gently lean forward.
GENERAL

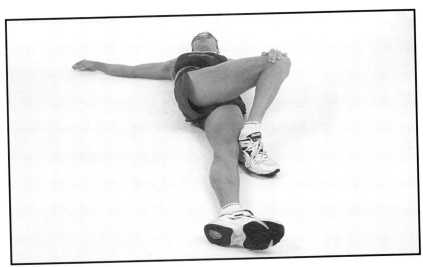

Fig 10.44 Lie on your back. Cross one leg over the other. Bring your foot up to your opposite knee. With your opposite arm pull your raised knee towards the ground.
GENERAL

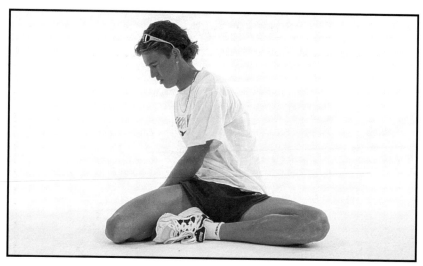

Fig 10.45 Sit with one leg crossed and your other leg behind your buttocks. Lean your whole body towards the leg that is behind your buttocks.

INTERMEDIATE

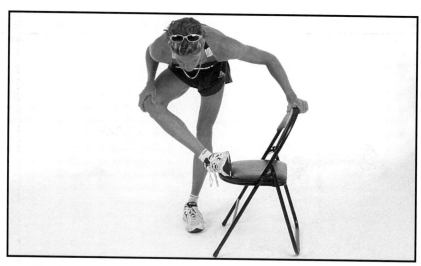

Fig 10.46 Stand beside a chair or table. Place the foot furthest from the object onto the object. Relax your leg, lean forward and bend your other leg, lowering yourself towards the ground. **INTERMEDIATE**

9. QUADRICEPS

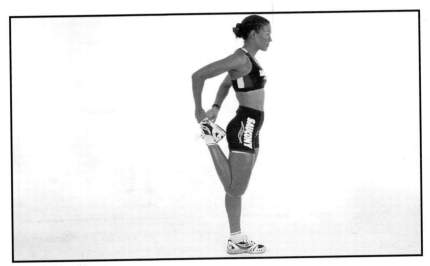

Fig 10.47 *Stand upright. Balance on one leg. Pull your other foot up behind your buttocks. Keep your knees together and push your hips forward. Hold on to something for balance.* **GENERAL**

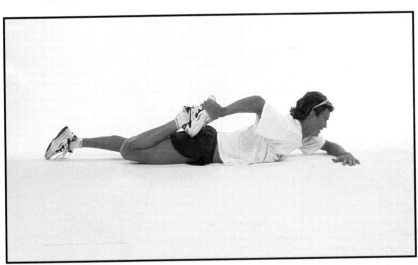

Fig 10.48 *Lie face down. Pull one foot up behind your buttocks. Keep your knees together and slowly raise your leg off the ground.* **GENERAL**

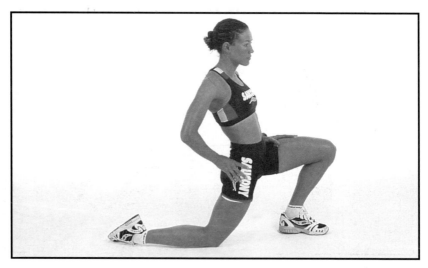

Fig 10.49 Kneel on one foot and the other knee. If needed, hold on to something to keep your balance. Push your hips forward.   ***GENERAL***

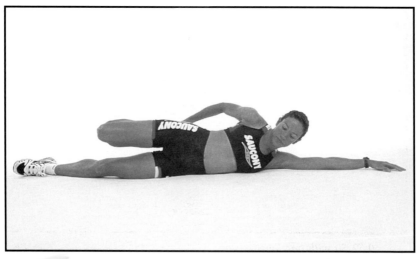

Fig 10.50 Lie on your side. Pull your top leg behind your buttocks. Keep your knees together. Push your hips forward.   ***GENERAL***

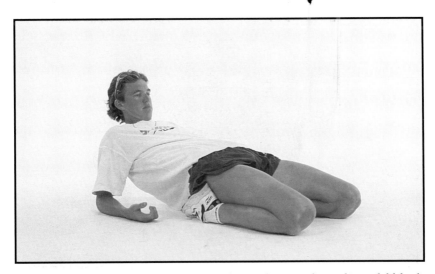

*Fig 10.51 Sit on the ground. Fold one leg under your buttocks or fold both legs under your buttocks. Slowly lean backwards. **Do not** attempt this stretch if you have, or are susceptible to, knee problems.*   ***ADVANCED***

10. BUTTOCKS

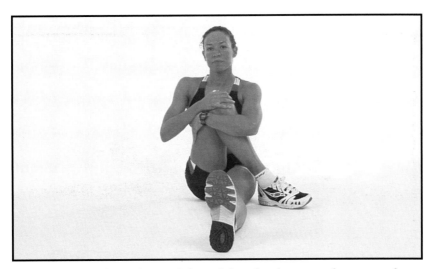

Fig 10.52 Sit with one leg straight and the other leg crossed over your knee. Pull the raised knee towards your opposite shoulder. Keep your back straight and your shoulders facing forward.   ***GENERAL***

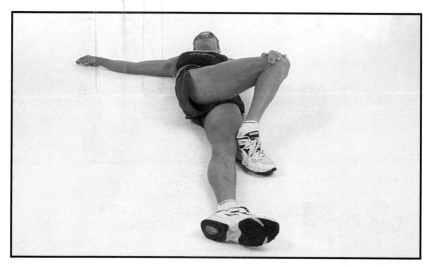

Fig 10.53 Lie on your back. Cross one leg over the other and raise your knee. Use your opposite hand to pull the raised knee towards the ground. Keep your hips on the ground. **GENERAL**

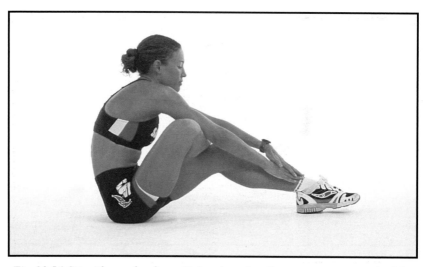

Fig 10.54 Sit with one leg bent. Raise the other foot up onto your raised leg and rest it on your thigh. Slowly lean forward. **GENERAL**

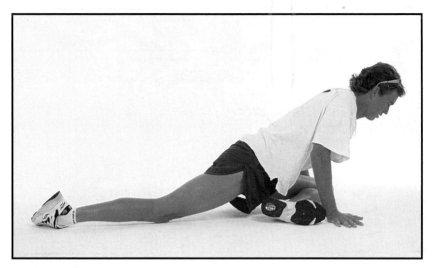

Fig 10.55 Lie on your stomach. Bend one leg under your stomach. Lean towards the ground. **INTERMEDIATE**

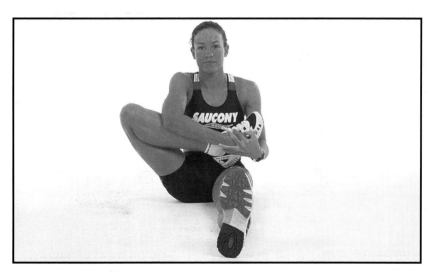

Fig 10.56 Sit with one leg straight. Hold your other ankle. Pull it directly towards your chest. **INTERMEDIATE**

11. HAMSTRINGS

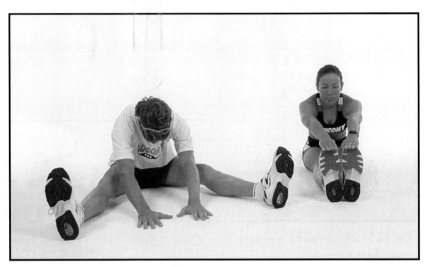

Fig 10.57 Sit with both legs straight out in front or at 45 degrees apart. Keep your toes pointing straight up. Make sure your back is straight. Reach forward. **GENERAL**

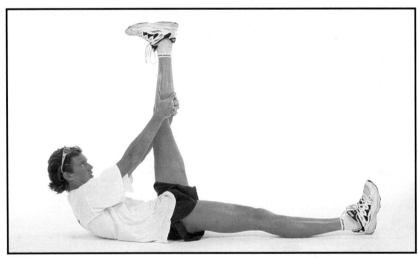

Fig 10.58 Lie on your back. Bend one leg. Raise your straight leg. Pull your leg towards your chest. **GENERAL**

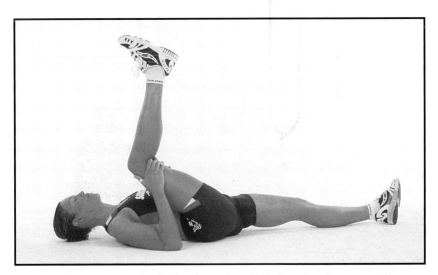

Fig 10.59 Lie on your back. Bend one leg. Pull the other knee towards your chest. Slowly and gently straighten your raised leg. **GENERAL**

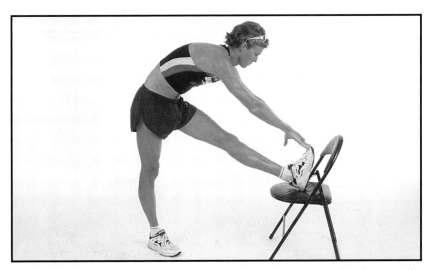

Fig 10.60 Stand upright. Raise one leg on to an object. Keep that leg straight and your toes pointing upwards. Lean forward. Keep your back straight. Reach towards your toes. **GENERAL**

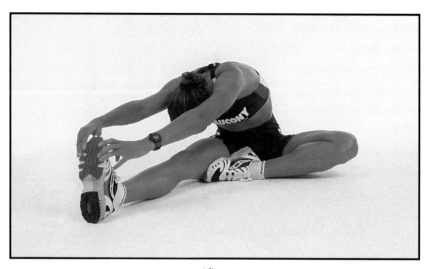

Fig 10.61 Sit with one leg straight out in front and toes pointing upwards. Bring your other foot towards your knee. Let your head fall forward. Reach towards your toes with both hands. **GENERAL**

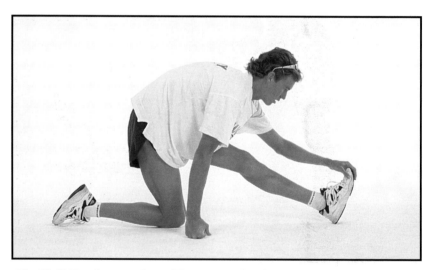

Fig 10.62 Kneel on one knee. Place your other leg straight forward with your heel on the ground. Keep your back straight. Point your toes towards your body. Reach towards your toes with one hand. **GENERAL**

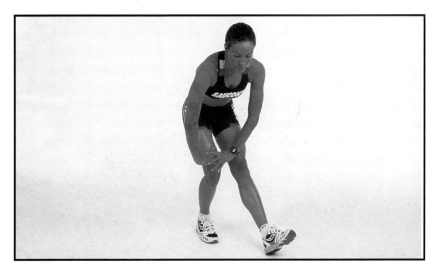

Fig 10.63 Stand with one knee bent and the other leg straight out in front. Point your toes towards your body. Lean forward. Keep your back straight. Rest your hands on your bent knee. **GENERAL**

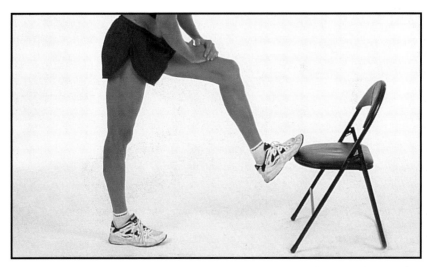

Fig 10.64 Stand with one foot raised onto a chair or an object. Keep your leg slightly bent. Let your heel drop off the edge of the object. Keep your back straight. Move your chest towards your thigh. **GENERAL**

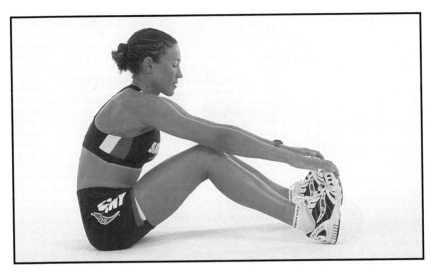

Fig 10.65 Sit on the ground with your legs slightly bent. Hold onto your toes with your hands. Pull your toes towards your body. Lean forward. Keep your back straight. **GENERAL**

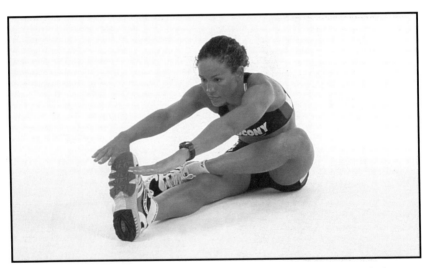

Fig 10.66 Sit with one leg straight out in front. Keep your toes pointing up. Cross your other leg over and rest your foot on your thigh. Lean forward. Keep your back straight. Reach for your toes. **INTERMEDIATE**

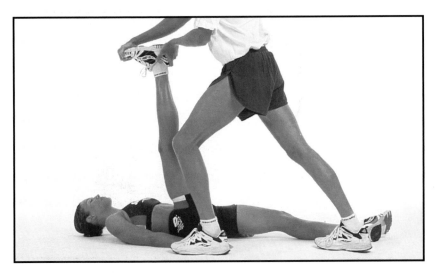

Fig 10.67 Lie on your back. Keep both legs straight. Have a partner raise one of your legs off the ground and as far back as is comfortable. Make sure your toes are pointing directly backwards.   ***INTERMEDIATE***

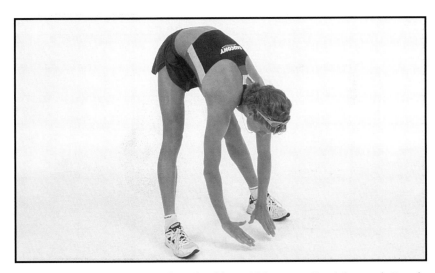

*Fig 10.68 Stand with your feet shoulder width apart. Bend forward. Reach towards the ground. **Do not** attempt this stretch if you have, or are susceptible to, back pain or back injury.*   ***ADVANCED***

12. ADDUCTORS

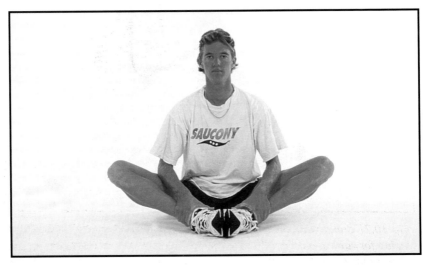

Fig 10.69 Sit with the soles of your feet together. Bring your feet towards your groin. Hold onto your ankles. Push your knee towards the ground with your elbows. Keep your back straight and upright.　　　**GENERAL**

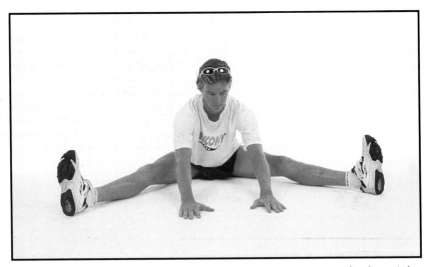

Fig 10.70 Sit with your legs straight and wide apart. Keep your back straight. Lean forward.　　　**GENERAL**

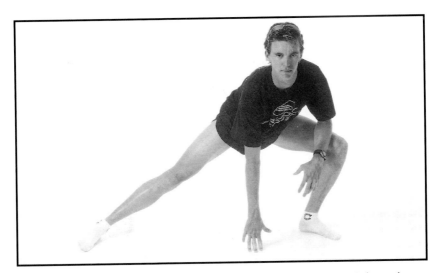

Fig 10.71 Stand with your feet wide apart. Keep one leg straight and toes facing forward. Bend the other leg and turn your toes out to the side. Lower your groin towards the ground. Rest your hands on the bent knee or the ground. **GENERAL**

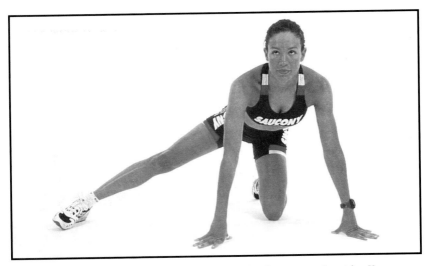

Fig 10.72 Kneel on one knee. Place your other leg out to the side. Keep your toes facing forward. Rest your hands on the ground. Slowly move your foot further out to the side. **GENERAL**

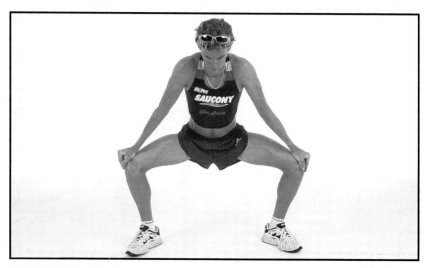

Fig 10.73 Stand with your feet wide apart and your toes pointing diagonally outwards. Bend at the knees, lean forward and use your hands to push your knees outwards. ***GENERAL***

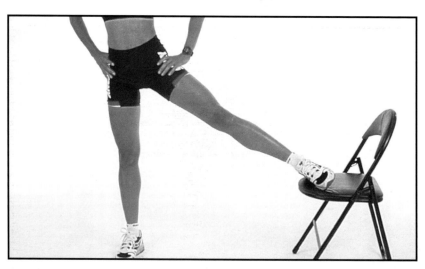

Fig 10.74 Stand upright. Place one leg out to the side and your foot up on a raised object. Keep your toes facing forward. Slowly move your other leg away from the object. ***INTERMEDIATE***

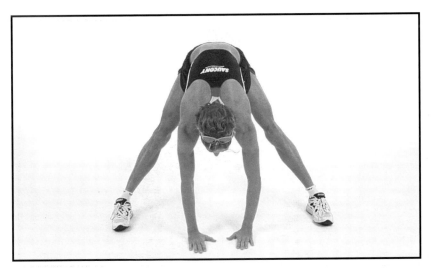

Fig 10.75 Stand with your feet wide apart and your toes facing forward. Lean forward. Reach towards the ground. **Do not** *attempt this stretch if you have, or are susceptible to back pain or back injury.* **ADVANCED**

13. ABDUCTORS

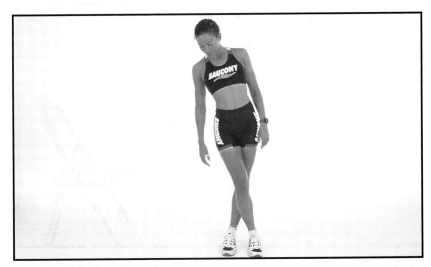

Fig 10.76 Stand upright. Cross one foot behind the other. Lean towards the foot that is behind the other. **GENERAL**

14. SHINS

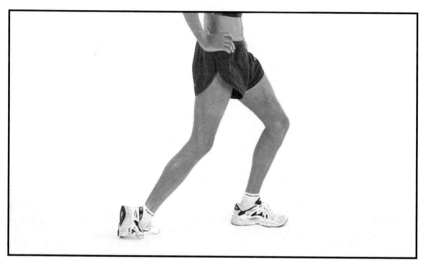

Fig 10.77 Stand upright. Place the top of your toes on the ground behind you. Push your ankle to the ground. **GENERAL**

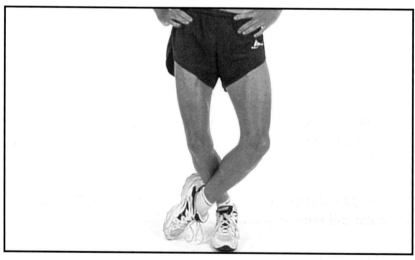

Fig 10.78 Stand upright. Place the top of your toes on the ground in front of your other foot. Slowly bend your other leg to force your ankle to the ground.
GENERAL

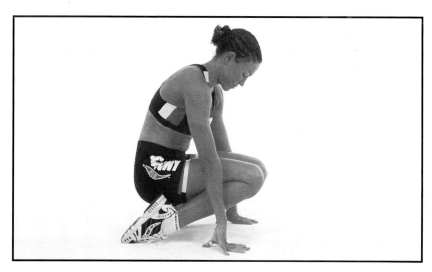

*Fig 10.79 Sit with your knees and feet flat on the ground. Sit back on your ankles. Keep your heals and knees together. Place your hands next to your knees. Slowly lean backwards. Raise your knees off the ground. **Do not** attempt this stretch if you have, or are susceptible to, knee or ankle problems.*

ADVANCED

15. CALVES

There are two separate parts to the calf muscle. To stretch them both properly we have to do a series of different stretches for both of the two separate parts.

The first part, the gastrocnemius, is the bulky mass situated at the top of the calf muscle, just below and behind the knee.

The other part is called the soleous, and it is situated lower in the calf area. It starts below and behind the knee and connects to the Achilles tendon at the back of the ankle.

GASTROCNEMIUS

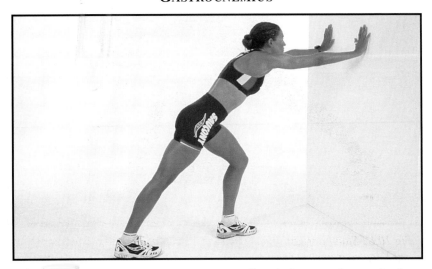

Fig 10.80 Stand upright. Lean against a wall and place one foot as far from the wall as is comfortable. Make sure that both toes are facing forward and your heel is on the ground. Keep your back leg straight. Lean towards the wall.   **GENERAL**

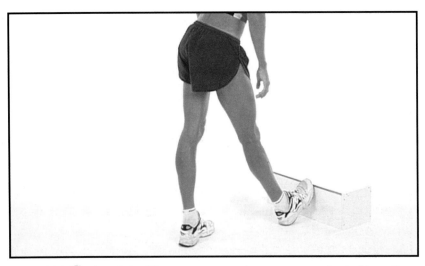

Fig 10.81 Stand upright. Place your toe against a step or raised object. Keep your leg straight. Lean towards your toe.   **GENERAL**

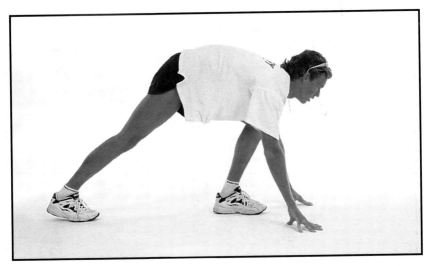

Fig 10.82 Stand upright. Place one foot in front of the other. Bend your front leg. Keep your back leg straight. Push your heal to the ground. Lean forward. Place your hands on the ground in front of you.　　　**GENERAL**

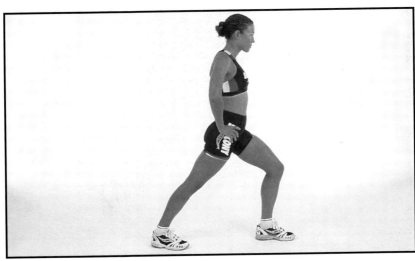

Fig 10.83 Stand upright. Take one big step backwards. Keep your back leg straight. Push your heel to the ground.　　　**GENERAL**

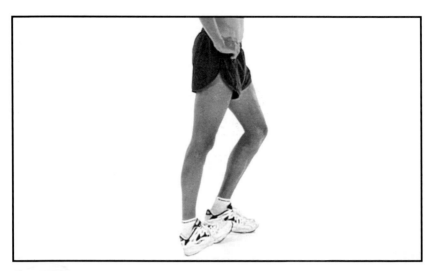

Fig 10.84 Stand on a raised object or step. Put the toes of one foot on the edge of the step. Keep your leg straight. Let your heal drop towards the ground.
GENERAL

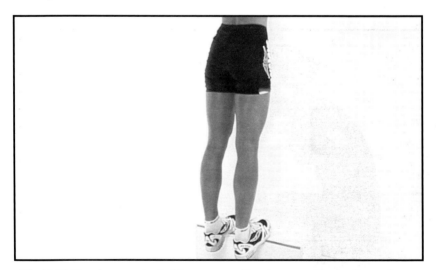

Fig 10.85 Stand on a raised object or step. Put the toes of both of your feet on the edge of the step. Keep your legs straight. Let your heals drop towards the ground. Lean forward. Place your hands in front of you. **GENERAL**

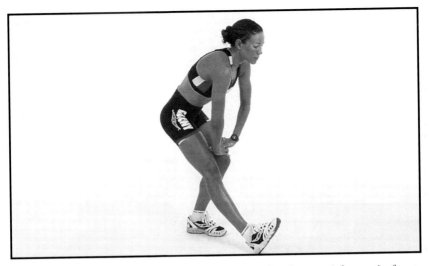

Fig 10.86 Stand with one knee bent and the other leg straight out in front. Point your toes towards your body. Lean forward. Keep your back straight. Rest your hands on your bent knee.   **GENERAL**

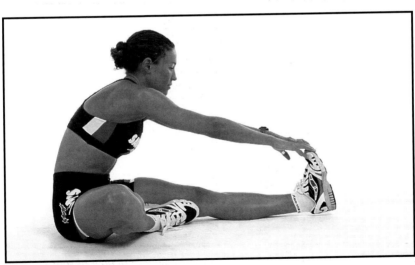

Fig 10.87 Sit with one leg straight and your toes pointing up. Lean forward. Pull your toes back towards your body.   **GENERAL**

SOLEOUS

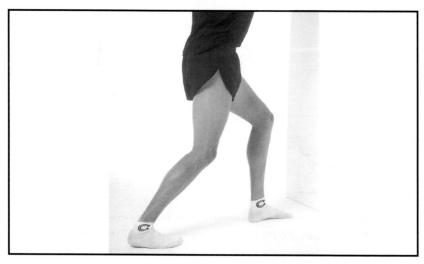

Fig 10.88 Stand upright. Lean against a wall and place one foot behind the other. Make sure that both toes are facing forward and your heel is on the ground. Bend your back leg. Lean towards the wall. **GENERAL**

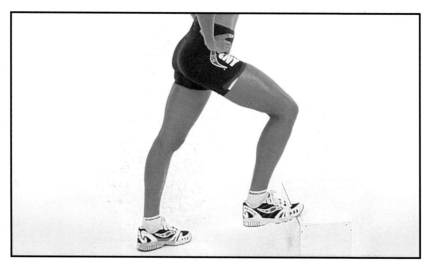

Fig 10.89 Stand upright. Place your toe against a step or raised object. Bend your leg. Lean towards your toe. **GENERAL**

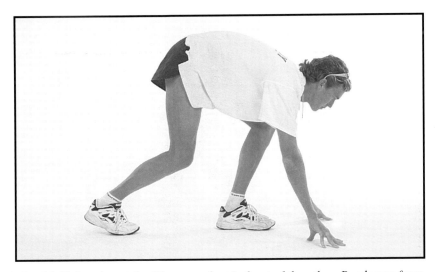

Fig 10.90 Stand upright. Place one foot in front of the other. Bend your front leg and your back leg. Push your back heel towards the ground. Lean forward placing your hands on the ground in front of you.   **GENERAL**

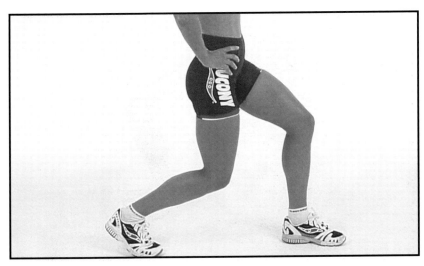

Fig 10.91 Stand upright. Take one big step backwards. Bend your back leg. Push your heel towards the ground.   **GENERAL**

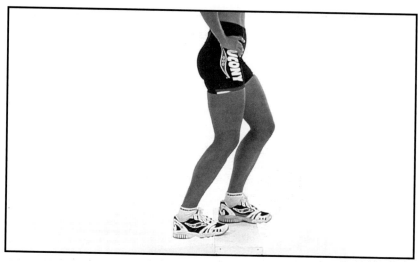

Fig 10.92 Stand on a raised object or step. Put the toes of one of your feet on the edge of the step. Bend your leg. Let your heal drop towards the ground.

GENERAL

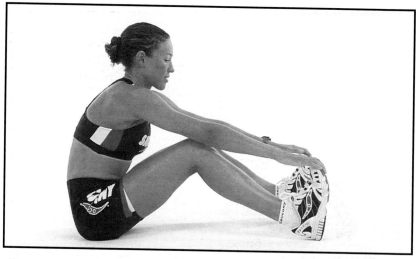

Fig 10.93 Sit with your legs out in front and bend both knees. Grab hold of your toes. Pull them towards your knees.

GENERAL

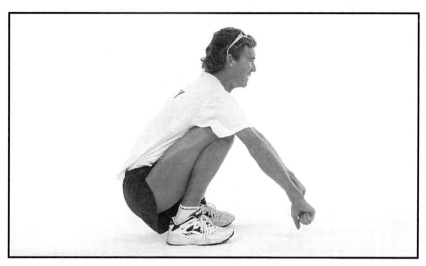

Fig 10.94 Stand with your feet at shoulder width apart. Bend your legs and lower to a sitting position. Place your hands on the ground in front.
INTERMEDIATE

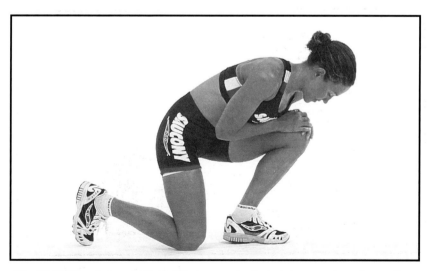

Fig 10.95 Kneel on one foot. Place your body weight over your knee. Keep your heel on the ground. Lean forward. **INTERMEDIATE**

16. ANKLES, FEET & TOES

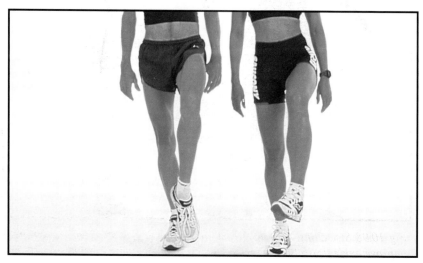

Fig 10.96 Raise one foot off the ground. Slowly rotate your foot in all directions. **GENERAL**

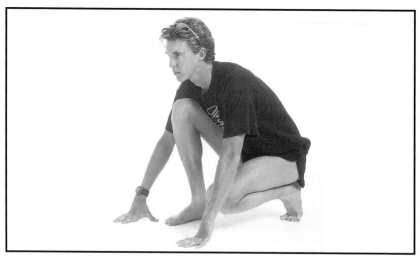

Fig 10.97 Kneel on one foot with your hands on the ground. Place your body weight over your knee and slowly move your knee towards the ground. Keep your toes on the ground and arch your foot. **GENERAL**

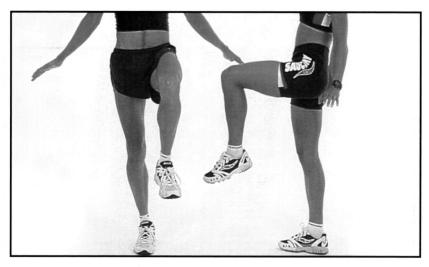

Fig 10.98 Stretching the muscles of your lower leg, (calves, shins) will help improve ankle flexibility. Another good practice to improve ankle strength are balancing exercises. Balance on one foot. Place your arms out to the side. Slowly move your upper body. **GENERAL**

17. WHOLE BODY

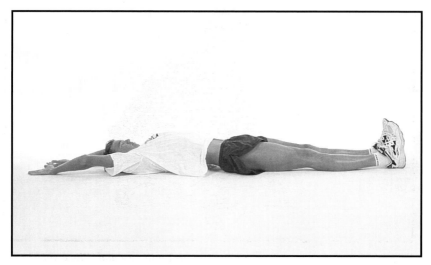

Fig 10.99 Lie on your back. Extend your arms behind you. Raise your toes. Now lengthen your body as much as you can. **GENERAL**